Dash Diet

Recipes

For Two

A Complete Cookbook: Tasty Low-Sodium Recipes To Improve Your Energy, Reduce Your Weight And Lower Your Blood Pressure

by Dash Diet Academy

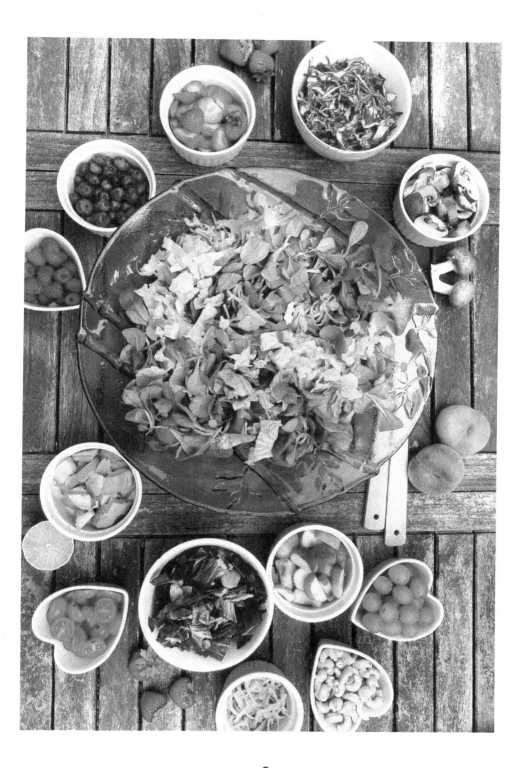

The following Book is reproduced below with the goal of providing information that is as accurate and reliable as possible. Regardless, purchasing this Book can be seen as consent to the fact that both the publisher and the author of this book are in no way experts on the topics discussed within and that any recommendations or suggestions that are made herein are for entertainment purposes only. Professionals should be consulted as needed prior to undertaking any of the action endorsed herein.

This declaration is deemed fair and valid by both the American Bar Association and the Committee of Publishers Association and is legally binding throughout the United States.

Furthermore, the transmission, duplication, or reproduction of any of the following work including specific information will be considered an illegal act irrespective of if it is done electronically or in print. This extends to creating a secondary or tertiary copy of the work or a recorded copy and is only allowed with the express written consent from the Publisher. All additional right reserved.

The information in the following pages is broadly considered a truthful and accurate account of facts and as such, any inattention, use, or misuse of the information in question by the reader will render any resulting actions solely under their purview. There are no scenarios in which the publisher or the original author of this work can be in any fashion deemed liable for any hardship or damages that may befall them after undertaking information described herein.

Additionally, the information in the following pages is intended only for informational purposes and should thus be thought of as universal. As befitting its nature, it is presented without assurance regarding its prolonged validity or interim quality. Trademarks that are mentioned are done without written consent and can in no way be considered an endorsement from the trademark holder.

Table of Content:

Introduction

DASH, initially, stand for Dietary Approaches to Stop Hypertension. However, over time, it has been expanded to Dietary Approaches to Stop Hypertension with the addition of heart healthy food options.

The diet helps in shrinking the waistline and improving the heart health. Proper implementation of the diet can lead to several health benefits, including lowering the risk of heart attack, stroke and the chances of developing type 2 diabetes. People who are suffering from diabetes are more susceptible to have a heart attack or stroke, especially if they are on high blood pressure medications. The same also applies to the high cholesterol levels in the blood. People who are suffering from high levels of cholesterol are at risk of developing heart disease. With the help of the DASH diet and the subsequent reduction in the cholesterol levels, the risk of developing heart disease is reduced to a great amount.

In the beginning, the DASH diet was only aimed to help the high blood pressure patients. Over time, the DASH diet has gained popularity among the general population. The reason for its growing popularity is the fact that more and more studies have proven its effectiveness. The DASH diet has proved to be so effective that it has been reported that the sodium levels in the diet affected the cardiovascular diseases.

The DASH diet has proven to be equally effective in both men and women. The main ingredient in the diet is the reduction in the amount of sodium and total daily intake of calories.

Changes in the blood pressure, as a result of the diet change, have been effectively proven by researchers. A study that was conducted at the John Hopkins University Medical Center provided high blood pressure patients with meals that included as much as 6 grams of salt. However, the blood pressure levels dropped down to a significant level in just four weeks. This study, along with many other studies suggested that there is a strong relationship between the amount of sodium in the diet and the blood pressure levels.

Dash Diet Plan

The ingredients in the following recipes are simple and common and they should not be substituted. The DASH diet is based on the suggested intake of the U.S. Department of Agriculture.

The standard DASH diet follows the recommendations of the Dietary Guidelines of Americans by which the daily sodium intake should be less than 2300 mg a day, which corresponds to 5 grams of sea salt (slightly less than a teaspoon, that measures approximately 5,9 grams).

The America Hearth Association sets the limit for an adult to 1500 mg a day, but the average American consumes more than the double of this recommended quantity: 3400 mg per day.

In both cases, the average quantity consumed per person is a lot higher than recommended, so you can see by yourself why an important change in food habits is so relevant to improve everyday life and personal health.

The recipes in this book show ingredients for two so it will be easy for you to half them if you cook just for yourself or double them up if you cook for a bigger family. They also include nutritional indications, which you may find helpful. The recipes are also very easy and quick, so all you need to do is start cooking and stop buying ready meals. Salt is largely used to preserve food, so ready made meals are VERY rich on it, to last longer. This is the reason why is so important you start to cook your own food from fresh ingredients, so you can consciously choose what is best for you and your family.

You will find out that you will rarely use red meat (which is not considered very hearth healthy) and the use of salt and savory food will be very limited. On the other hand you will season your dishes with a lot of amazing spices and aromatic plants that will enhance your foods flavor; you will also be using a very vide range of fresh vegetables that will really make your dishes deliciously tasty.

If you are ready, we can start cooking!

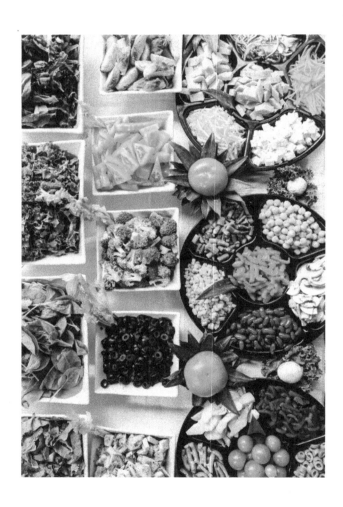

Breakfast

Roasted Feta with Kale and Lemon Yogurt

Preparation Time: 15 Minutes

Cooking Time: 20 Minutes

Servings: 2

Ingredients:

- 1 tablespoon extra-virgin olive oil

- 1 onion, julienned

- ¼ teaspoon kosher salt

- 1 teaspoon ground turmeric

- ½ teaspoon ground cumin

- ½ teaspoon ground coriander

- ¼ teaspoon freshly ground black pepper

- 1 bunch kale, stemmed and chopped

- 7-ounce block feta cheese, cut into ¼-inch-thick slices

- ½ cup plain Greek yogurt

- 1 tablespoon lemon juice

Directions:

1. Preheat the oven to 400°F.

2. Heat the olive oil in a large ovenproof skillet or sauté pan over medium heat. Add the onion and salt; sauté until lightly golden brown, about 5 minutes. Add the turmeric, cumin, coriander, and black pepper; sauté for 30 seconds. Add the kale and sauté about 2 minutes. Add ½ cup water and continue to cook down the kale, about 3 minutes.

3. Remove from the heat and place the feta cheese slices on top of the kale mixture. Place in the oven and bake until the feta softens, 10 to 12 minutes.

4. In a small bowl, combine the yogurt and lemon juice.

5. Serve the kale and feta cheese topped with the lemon yogurt.

Nutrition: Calories: 210; Total fat: 14g; Saturated fat: 8g; Cholesterol: 44mg; Sodium: 565mg; Potassium: 340mg; Total Carbohydrates: 11g; Fiber: 2g; Sugars: 5g; Protein: 11g; Magnesium: 55mg; Calcium: 375mg

Baked Falafel Sliders

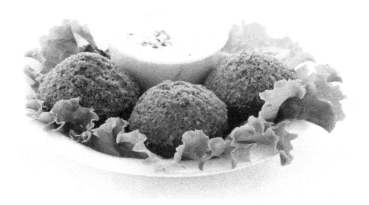

Preparation Time: 10 Minutes

Cooking Time: 30 Minutes

Servings: 2

Ingredients:

- 1 (15-ounce) can no-salt-added or low-sodium chickpeas, drained and rinsed

- 1 onion, roughly chopped

- 2 garlic cloves, peeled

- 2 tablespoons fresh parsley, chopped

- 2 tablespoons whole-wheat flour

- ½ teaspoon ground coriander

- ½ teaspoon ground cumin

- ½ teaspoon baking powder

- ¼ teaspoon freshly ground black pepper

- Olive oil cooking spray

Directions:

1. Preheat the oven to 350°F. Line a baking sheet with parchment paper or foil and lightly spray with olive oil cooking spray.

2. In a food processor, add the chickpeas, onion, garlic, parsley, flour, coriander, cumin, baking powder, and black pepper. Process until smooth, stopping to scrape down the sides of the bowl.

3. Make 6 slider patties, each with a heaping ¼ cup of mixture, and arrange on the prepared baking sheet. Bake for 30 minutes, turning over halfway through.

Nutrition: Calories: 90; Total fat: 1g; Saturated fat: 0g; Cholesterol: 0mg; Sodium: 110mg; Potassium: 230mg; Total Carbohydrates: 17g; Fiber: 3g; Sugars: 1g; Protein: 4g; Magnesium: 28mg; Calcium: 62mg

Healthy Cucumber Soup

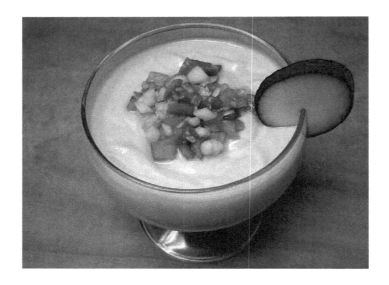

Preparation Time: 14 Minutes

Cooking Time: 0 Minutes

Servings: 2

Ingredients:

- 2 tablespoons garlic, minced

- 4 cups English cucumbers, peeled and diced

- ½ cup onions, diced

- 1 tablespoon lemon juice

- 1 ½ cups vegetable broth

- ½ teaspoon sunflower seeds

- ¼ teaspoon red pepper flakes

- ¼ cup parsley, diced

- ½ cup Greek yogurt, plain

Directions:

1. Add the listed ingredients to a blender and blend to emulsify (keep aside ½ cup of chopped cucumbers).

2. Blend until smooth.

3. Divide the soup amongst 4 servings and top with extra cucumbers.

4. Enjoy chilled!

Nutrition:

Calories: 371 , Fat: 36g

Carbohydrates: 8g, Protein: 4g

Coconut Avocado Soup

Preparation Time: 5 minutes

Cooking Time: 5-10 minutes

Servings: 2

Ingredients:

- 2 cups vegetable stock

- 2 teaspoons Thai green curry paste

- Pepper as needed

- 1 avocado, chopped

- 1 tablespoon cilantro, chopped

- Lime wedges

- 1 cup coconut milk

Directions:

1. Add milk, avocado, curry paste, pepper to blender and blend.

2. Take a pan and place it over medium heat.

3. Add mixture and heat, simmer for 5 minutes.

4. Stir in seasoning, cilantro and simmer for 1 minute.

5. Serve and enjoy!

Nutrition:

Calories: 250

Fat: 30g

Net Carbohydrates: 2g

Protein: 4g

Chickpeas and Kale with Spicy Pomodoro Sauce

Preparation Time: 10 Minutes

Cooking Time: 35 Minutes

Servings: 2

Ingredients:

- 2 tablespoons extra-virgin olive oil

- 4 garlic cloves, sliced

- 1 teaspoon red pepper flakes

- 1 (28-ounce) can no-salt-added crushed tomatoes

- ½ teaspoon honey

- 1 bunch kale, stemmed and chopped

- 2 (15-ounce) cans no-salt-added or low-sodium chickpeas, drained and rinsed

- ¼ cup fresh basil, chopped

- ¼ cup grated pecorino Romano cheese

Directions:

1. Heat the olive oil in a large skillet or sauté pan over medium heat then add the garlic and red pepper flakes and sauté until the garlic is a light golden brown, about 2 minutes. Add the tomatoes, and honey and mix well. Reduce the heat to low and simmer for 20 minutes.

2. Add the kale and mix in well. Cook about 5 minutes. Add the chickpeas and simmer about 5 minutes.

3. Remove from heat and stir in the basil. Serve topped with pecorino cheese.

Nutrition: Calories: 420; Total fat: 13g; Saturated fat: 4g; Cholesterol: 15mg; Sodium: 570mg; Potassium: 1,250mg; Total Carbohydrates: 54g; Fiber: 12g; Sugars: 9g; Protein: 20g; Magnesium: 175mg; Calcium: 440mg

Coconut Arugula Soup

Preparation Time: 5 minutes

Cooking Time: 5-10 minutes

Servings: 2

Ingredients:

- Black pepper as needed

- 1 tablespoon olive oil

- 2 tablespoons chives, chopped

- 2 garlic cloves, minced

- 10 ounces baby arugula

- 2 tablespoons tarragon, chopped

- 4 tablespoons coconut milk yogurt

- 6 cups chicken stock

- 2 tablespoons mint, chopped

- 1 onion, chopped

- ½ cup coconut milk

Directions:

1. Take a saucepan and place it over medium-high heat, add oil and let it heat up.

2. Add onion and garlic and fry for 5 minutes.

3. Stir in stock and coconut milk and reduce the heat, let it simmer.

4. Stir in tarragon, arugula, mint, parsley and cook for 6 minutes.

5. Mix in seasoning, chives, coconut yogurt and serve.

6. Enjoy!

Nutrition:

Calories: 180

Fat: 14g

Net Carbohydrates: 20g

Protein: 2g

Ginger Zucchini Avocado Soup

Preparation Time: 7 minutes

Cooking Time: 25 minutes

Servings: 2

Ingredients:

- 1 red bell pepper, chopped

- 1 big avocado

- 1 teaspoon ginger, grated

- Pepper as needed

- 2 tablespoons avocado oil

- 4 scallions, chopped

- 1 tablespoon lemon juice

- 29 ounces vegetable stock

- 1 garlic clove, minced

- 2 zucchini, chopped

- 1 cup water

Directions:

1. Take a pan and place over medium heat, add onion and fry for 3 minutes.

2. Stir in ginger, garlic and cook for 1 minute.

3. Mix in seasoning, zucchini stock, water and boil for 10 minutes.

4. Remove soup from fire and let it sit, blend in avocado and blend using an immersion blender.

5. Heat over low heat for about 10 more minutes.

6. Adjust your seasoning and add lemon juice and bell pepper.

7. Serve and enjoy!

Nutrition:

Calories: 155

Fat: 11g

Carbohydrates: 10g

Protein: 7g

Ricotta, Basil, and Pistachio–Stuffed Zucchini

Preparation Time: 15 Minutes

Cooking Time: 25 Minutes

Servings: 2

Ingredients:

- 2 medium zucchini, halved lengthwise

- 1 tablespoon extra-virgin olive oil

- 1 onion, diced

- 2 garlic cloves, minced

- ¾ cup ricotta cheese

- ¼ cup unsalted pistachios, shelled and chopped

- ¼ cup fresh basil, chopped

- 1 large egg, beaten

- ¼ teaspoon freshly ground black pepper

Directions:

1. Preheat the oven to 425°F. Line a baking sheet with parchment paper or foil.

2. Scoop out the seeds/pulp from the zucchini, leaving ¼-inch flesh around the edges. Transfer the pulp to a cutting board and chop the pulp.

3. Heat the olive oil in a large skillet or sauté pan over medium heat.

4. Add the onion, and the pulp, and sauté about 5 minutes. Add the garlic and sauté 30 seconds.

5. In a medium bowl, combine the ricotta cheese, pistachios, basil, egg, and black pepper. Add the onion mixture and mix together well.

6. Place the 4 zucchini halves on the prepared baking sheet. Fill the zucchini halves with the ricotta mixture. Bake for 20 minutes, or until golden brown.

Nutrition: Calories: 200; Total fat: 12g; Saturated fat: 4g; Cholesterol: 61mg; Sodium: 360mg; Potassium: 650mg; Total Carbohydrates: 14g; Fiber: 3g; Sugars: 7g; Protein: 11g; Magnesium: 52mg; Calcium: 185mg

Lunch

Pasta & CO. Ideas

Pistachio Mint Pesto Pasta

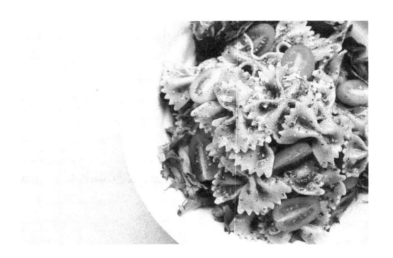

Preparation Time: 10 Minutes

Cooking Time: 10 Minutes

Servings: 2

Ingredients:

- 8 ounces whole-wheat pasta

- 1 cup fresh mint

- ½ cup fresh basil

- ⅓ cup unsalted pistachios, shelled

- 1 garlic clove, peeled

- Juice of ½ lime

- ⅓ cup extra-virgin olive oil

Directions:

1. Cook the pasta according to the package directions(except for salt and oil). Drain, reserving ½ cup of the pasta water, and set aside.

2. In a food processor, add the mint, basil, pistachios, garlic, and lime juice. Process until the pistachios are coarsely ground. Add the olive oil in a slow, steady stream and process until incorporated.

3. In a large bowl, mix the pasta with the pistachio pesto; toss well to incorporate. If a thinner, saucier consistency is desired, add some of the reserved pasta water and toss well.

Nutrition: Calories: 420; Total fat: 3g; Saturated fat: 3g; Cholesterol: 0mg; Sodium: 150mg; Potassium: 290mg; Total Carbohydrates: 48g; Fiber: 2g; Sugars: 1g; Protein: 11g; Magnesium: 100mg; Calcium: 65mg

Burst Cherry Tomato Sauce with Angel Hair Pasta

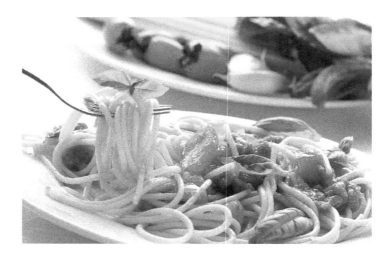

Preparation Time: 10 Minutes

Cooking Time: 20 Minutes

Servings: 2

Ingredients:

- 8 ounces angel hair pasta

- 2 tablespoons extra-virgin olive oil

- 3 garlic cloves, minced

- 3 pints cherry tomatoes

- ¼ teaspoon red pepper flakes

- ¾ cup fresh basil, chopped

- 1 tablespoon white balsamic vinegar (optional)

- ¼ cup grated Parmesan cheese (optional)

Directions:

1. Cook the pasta according to the package directions (except for salt and oil). Drain and set aside.

2. Heat the olive oil in a skillet or large sauté pan over medium-high heat. Add the garlic and sauté for 30 seconds. Add the tomatoes, and red pepper flakes and cook, stirring occasionally, until the tomatoes burst, about 15 minutes.

3. Remove from the heat and add the pasta and basil. Toss together well. (For out-of-season tomatoes, add the vinegar, if desired, and mix well.)

4. Serve with the grated Parmesan cheese, if desired.

Nutrition: Calories: 305; Total fat: 8g; Saturated fat: 1g; Cholesterol: 0mg; Sodium: 155mg; Potassium: 690mg; Total Carbohydrates: 53g; Fiber: 3g; Sugars: 7g; Protein: 11g; Magnesium: 112mg; Calcium: 65mg

Farro with Roasted Tomatoes and Mushrooms

Preparation Time: 20 Minutes

Cooking Time: 1 Hour

Servings: 2

Ingredients:

FOR THE TOMATOES

- 2 pints cherry tomatoes

- 1 teaspoon extra-virgin olive oil

FOR THE FARRO

- 3 to 4 cups water

- ½ cup farro

FOR THE MUSHROOMS

- 2 tablespoons extra-virgin olive oil

- 1 onion, julienned

- ¼ teaspoon freshly ground black pepper

- 10 ounces baby bella (crimini) mushrooms, stemmed and sliced thin

- ½ cup no-salt-added vegetable stock

- 1 (15-ounce) can no-salt-added or low-sodium cannellini beans, drained and rinsed

- 1 cup baby spinach

- 2 tablespoons fresh basil, cut into ribbons

- ¼ cup pine nuts, toasted

- Aged balsamic vinegar (optional)

Directions:

TO MAKE THE TOMATOES

Preheat the oven to 400°F. Line a baking sheet with parchment paper or foil. Toss the tomatoes and olive oil together on the baking sheet and roast for 30 minutes.

TO MAKE THE FARRO

Bring the water and farro to a boil in a medium saucepan or pot over high heat. Cover, reduce the heat to low, and simmer, and cook for 30 minutes, or until the farro is al dente. Drain and set aside.

TO MAKE THE MUSHROOMS

1. Heat the olive oil in a large skillet or sauté pan over medium-low heat. Add the onions, and black pepper and sauté until golden brown and starting to caramelize, about 15 minutes. Add the mushrooms, increase the heat to medium, and sauté until the liquid has evaporated and the mushrooms brown, about 10 minutes. Add the vegetable stock and deglaze the pan, scraping up any brown bits, and reduce the liquid for about 5 minutes. Add the beans and warm through, about 3 minutes.

2. Remove from the heat and mix in the spinach, basil, pine nuts, roasted tomatoes, and farro. Garnish with a drizzle of balsamic vinegar, if desired.

Nutrition: Calories: 375; Total fat: 15g; Saturated fat: 2g; Cholesterol: 0mg; Sodium: 305mg; Potassium: 1,050mg; Total Carbohydrates: 48g; Fiber: 10g; Sugars: 8g; Protein: 14g; Magnesium: 110mg; Calcium: 100mg

Baked Orzo with Eggplant, Swiss Chard, and Mozzarella

Preparation Time: 20 Minutes

Cooking Time: 1 Hour

Servings: 2

Ingredients:

- 2 tablespoons extra-virgin olive oil

- 1 large (1-pound) eggplant, diced small

- 2 carrots, peeled and diced small

- 2 celery stalks, diced small

- 1 onion, diced small

- 3 garlic cloves, minced

- ¼ teaspoon freshly ground black pepper

- 1 cup whole-wheat orzo

- 1 teaspoon no-salt-added tomato paste

- 1½ cups no-salt-added vegetable stock

- 1 cup Swiss chard, stemmed and chopped small

- 2 tablespoons fresh oregano, chopped

- Zest of 1 lemon

- 4 ounces mozzarella cheese, diced small

- ¼ cup grated Parmesan cheese

- 2 tomatoes, sliced ½-inch-thick

Directions:

1. Preheat the oven to 400°F.

2. Heat the olive oil in a large oven-safe sauté pan over medium heat. Add the eggplant, carrots, celery, onion and sauté about 10 minutes. Add the garlic and black pepper and sauté about 30 seconds. Add the orzo and tomato paste and sauté 1 minute. Add the vegetable stock and deglaze the pan, scraping up the brown bits. Add the Swiss chard, oregano, and lemon zest and stir until the chard wilts.

3. Remove from the heat and mix in the mozzarella cheese. Smooth the top of the orzo mixture flat. Sprinkle the Parmesan cheese over the top. Arrange the tomatoes in a

single layer on top of the Parmesan cheese. Bake for 45 minutes.

Nutrition: Calories: 470; Total fat: 17g; Saturated fat: 6g; Cholesterol: 28mg; Sodium: 545mg; Potassium: 770mg; Total Carbohydrates: 65g; Fiber: 7g; Sugars: 13g; Protein: 18g; Magnesium: 53mg; Calcium: 270mg

Barley Risotto with Tomatoes

Preparation Time: 20 Minutes

Cooking Time: 45 Minutes

Servings: 2

Ingredients:

- 2 tablespoons extra-virgin olive oil

- 2 celery stalks, diced

- ½ cup shallots, diced

- 4 garlic cloves, minced

- 3 cups no-salt-added vegetable stock

- 1 (14.5-ounce) can no-salt-added diced tomatoes

- 1 (14.5-ounce) can no-salt-added crushed tomatoes

- 1 cup pearl barley

- Zest of 1 lemon

- ½ teaspoon smoked paprika

- ¼ teaspoon red pepper flakes

- ¼ teaspoon freshly ground black pepper

- 4 thyme sprigs

- 1 dried bay leaf

- 2 cups baby spinach

- ½ cup crumbled feta cheese

- 1 tablespoon fresh oregano, chopped

- 1 tablespoon fennel seeds, toasted (optional)

Directions:

1. Heat the olive oil in a large saucepan over medium heat. Add the celery and shallots and sauté, about 4 to 5 minutes. Add the garlic and sauté 30 seconds. Add the vegetable stock, diced tomatoes, crushed tomatoes, barley, lemon zest, paprika, red pepper flakes, black pepper, thyme, and the bay leaf, and mix well. Bring to a boil, then lower to low, and simmer. Cook, stirring occasionally, for 40 minutes.

2. Remove the bay leaf and thyme sprigs. Stir in the spinach.

3. In a small bowl, combine the feta, oregano, and fennel seeds. Serve the barley risotto in bowls topped with the feta mixture.

Nutrition: Calories: 375; Total fat: 12g; Saturated fat: 4g; Cholesterol: 17mg; Sodium: 570mg; Potassium: 850mg; Total Carbohydrates: 57g; Fiber: 13g; Sugars: 11g; Protein: 11g; Magnesium: 90mg; Calcium: 210mg

Shrimp & Broccoli with Angel Hair

Preparation Time: 10 Minutes

Cooking Time: 15 Minutes

Servings: 2

Ingredients:

- 4 teaspoons olive oil, divided

- 1 garlic clove, pressed or minced

- 1 broccoli head, cut into florets

- 12 frozen, cooked large shrimp, peeled, deveined, and tails removed

- 4 ounces angel hair pasta

- 2 tablespoons Parmesan cheese

- Freshly ground black pepper (optional)

Directions:

1. Fill a large stockpot three-quarters full with water and bring it to a boil over high heat.

2. Heat 1 teaspoon of oil in a medium skillet over medium-high heat. Add the garlic and cook for 1 minute. Add the broccoli and sauté for 3 to 4 minutes. Cover and let the vegetables steam for an additional 2 minutes. The broccoli should be bright green and fork-tender. Set aside off the heat.

3. Add the angel hair to the boiling water and cook for 2 to 4 minutes, according to the directions on the package (except for salt and oil). Drain and immediately add to the skillet. Add the remaining 1 tablespoon of olive oil and stir. Return to low heat to heat through, about 3 minutes.

4. Divide the pasta between two dishes and garnish with the Parmesan cheese and pepper to taste (if using).

Nutrition: Calories: 456; Total fat: 12g; Carbohydrates: 64g; Fiber: 10g; Protein: 25g; Calcium: 230mg; Sodium: 583mg; Potassium: 1158mg; Vitamin D: 0mcg; Iron: 4mg; Zinc: 3mg

Saucy Penne with Shrimp, Peas & Walnuts

Preparation Time: 5 Minutes

Cooking Time: 20 Minutes

Servings: 2

Ingredients:

- 1 teaspoon olive oil

- 12 large cooked frozen shrimp (peeled and deveined), thawed

- 1 cup frozen peas

- ½ cup chopped walnuts

- ½ teaspoon salt-free Italian seasoning blend

- 2 teaspoons unsalted butter

- 1 tablespoon all-purpose flour

- 1 cup 1 percent milk

- 2 tablespoons light cream cheese

- ¼ cup grated Parmesan cheese, divided

- 4 ounces penne pasta

- Freshly ground black pepper

Directions:

1. Fill a large stockpot three-quarters full with water and then bring it to a boil on high heat.

2. In a medium saucepan, heat the oil over medium-high heat and sauté the shrimp, peas, walnuts, and seasoning for 3 to 4 minutes. (Make sure any liquid from the shrimp is evaporated.) Transfer the mixture to a small bowl.

3. Wipe out the saucepan with a paper towel and melt the butter in it over medium heat. Whisk in the flour for 1 minute. Slowly pour in the milk and bring it to a boil, whisking occasionally. Reduce the heat to low, simmer, and stir in the cream cheese until it melts, about 3 minutes. Add 3 tablespoons of the Parmesan cheese and continue stirring until the sauce is creamy and well-blended, about 2 minutes. Add more milk if the sauce gets too thick. Remove it from the heat.

4. When the water is boiling, add the penne and boil for 8 to 9 minutes (or follow the package directions for al dente, but don't add oil or salt to your water).

5. Drain the pasta and add it to the sauce. Stir to combine. Transfer the pasta to a serving dish and top it with the shrimp mixture. Garnish the pasta with the remaining Parmesan cheese, season it with pepper, and serve.

Nutrition: Calories: 673; Total fat: 34g; Carbohydrates: 64g; Fiber: 6g; Protein: 31g; Calcium: 390mg; Sodium: 653mg; Potassium: 698mg; Vitamin D: 1mcg; Iron: 3mg; Zinc: 4mg

Angel Hair with Smoked Salmon & Asparagus

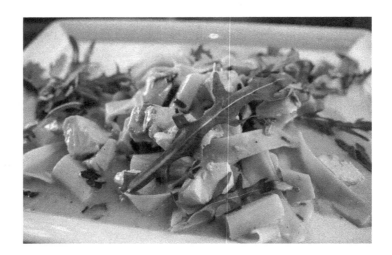

Preparation Time: 15 Minutes

Cooking Time: 15 Minutes

Servings: 2

Ingredients:

- 20 asparagus spears, trimmed and cut into 2-inch pieces

- 2 tablespoons olive oil, divided

- 4 ounces angel hair pasta

- 2 ounces smoked salmon, cut into bite-size pieces

- 1 teaspoon capers

- 2 tablespoons grated Parmesan cheese

- Freshly ground black pepper

Directions:

1. Fill a large stockpot three-quarters full with water and bring it to a boil over high heat.

2. Add 2 tablespoons of water to a large nonstick skillet over medium heat. When the water is simmering, add the asparagus, cover, and steam for 6 minutes. Remove the lid, drain off any remaining water, and add 1½ teaspoons oil and sauté for 1 to 2 more minutes.

3. Add the angel hair pasta to the boiling water and cook for 3 minutes (or according to the package directions). Drain the pasta, transfer it to a serving bowl, and add the asparagus, smoked salmon, the remaining 1½ tablespoons oil, and the capers and toss gently.

4. Serve topped with the Parmesan cheese and seasoned to taste with pepper.

Nutrition: Calories: 416; Total fat: 17g; Carbohydrates: 49g; Fiber: 5g; Protein: 18g; Calcium: 97mg; Sodium: 320mg; Potassium: 509mg; Vitamin D: 5mcg; Iron: 6mg; Zinc: 2mg

Soup Ideas

Mushroom Cream Soup

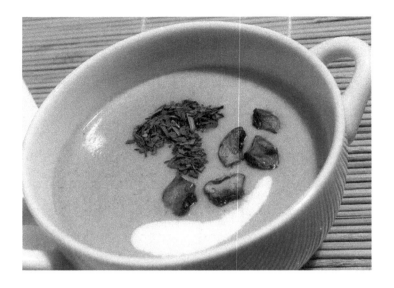

Preparation Time: 5 minutes

Cooking Time: 30 minutes

Servings: 2

Ingredients:

- 1 tablespoon olive oil

- ½ large onion, diced

- 20 ounces mushrooms, sliced

- 6 garlic cloves, minced

- 2 cups vegetable broth

- 1 cup coconut cream

- ¾ teaspoon sunflower seeds

- ¼ teaspoon black pepper

- 1 cup almond milk

Directions:

1. Take a large sized pot and place it over medium heat.

2. Add onion and mushrooms to the olive oil and sauté for 10-15 minutes.

3. Make sure to keep stirring it from time to time until browned evenly.

4. Add garlic and sauté for 10 minutes more.

5. Add vegetable broth, coconut cream, almond milk, black pepper and sunflower seeds.

6. Bring it to a boil and lower the temperature to low.

7. Simmer for 15 minutes.

8. Use an immersion blender to puree the mixture.

9. Enjoy!

Nutrition:

Calories: 200

Fat: 17g

Carbohydrates: 5g

Protein: 4g

Curious Roasted Garlic Soup

Preparation Time: 10 minutes

Cooking Time: 60 minutes

Servings: 2

Ingredients:

- 1 tablespoon olive oil

- 2 bulbs garlic, peeled

- 3 shallots, chopped

- 1 large head cauliflower, chopped

- 3 cups vegetable broth

- Sunflower seeds and pepper to taste

Directions:

1. Pre-heat your oven to 400 degrees F.

2. Slice ¼ inch top of garlic bulb and place it in aluminum foil.

3. Grease with olive oil and roast in oven for 35 minutes.

4. Squeeze flesh out of the roasted garlic.

5. Heat oil in saucepan and add shallots, sauté for 6 minutes.

6. Add garlic, cauliflower and broth.

7. Cover pan and reduce heat to low.

8. Let it cook for 15-20 minutes.

9. Use an immersion blender to puree the mixture.

10. Season soup with sunflower seeds and pepper.

11. Serve and enjoy!

Nutrition:

Calories: 142

Fat: 8g

Carbohydrates: 3.4g

Protein: 4g

Amazing Roasted Carrot Soup

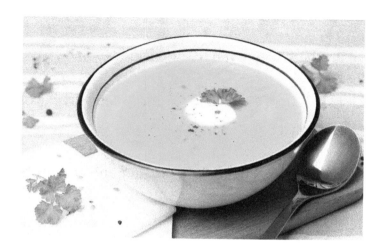

Preparation Time: 10 minutes

Cooking Time: 50 minutes

Servings: 2

Ingredients:

- 8 large carrots, washed and peeled

- 6 tablespoons olive oil

- 3 cups vegetable broth

- Cayenne pepper to taste

- Sunflower seeds and pepper to taste

Directions:

1. Pre-heat your oven to 425 degrees F.

2. Take a baking sheet and add carrots, drizzle olive oil and roast for 30-45 minutes.

3. Put roasted carrots into blender and add broth, puree.

4. Pour into saucepan and heat soup.

5. Season with sunflower seeds, pepper and cayenne.

6. Drizzle olive oil.

7. Serve and enjoy!

Nutrition:

Calories: 222

Fat: 18g

Net Carbohydrates: 7g

Protein: 5g

Awesome Cabbage Soup

Preparation Time: 7 minutes

Cooking Time: 25 minutes

Servings: 2

Ingredients:

- 3 cups non-fat beef stock

- 2 garlic cloves, minced

- 1 tablespoon tomato paste

- 2 cups cabbage, chopped

- ½ yellow onion

- ½ cup carrot, chopped

- ½ cup green beans

- ½ cup zucchini, chopped

- ½ teaspoon basil

- ½ teaspoon oregano

- Sunflower seeds and pepper as needed

Directions:

1. Grease a pot with non-stick cooking spray.

2. Place it over medium heat and allow the oil to heat up.

3. Add onions, carrots, and garlic and sauté for 5 minutes.

4. Add broth, tomato paste, green beans, cabbage, basil, oregano, sunflower seeds, and pepper.

5. Bring the whole mix to a boil and reduce the heat, simmer for 5-10 minutes until all veggies are tender.

6. Add zucchini and simmer for 5 minutes more.

7. Sever hot and enjoy!

Nutrition:

Calories: 22

Fat: 0g

Carbohydrates: 5g

Protein: 1g

Greek Lemon and Chicken Soup

Preparation Time: 15 minutes

Cooking Time: 30 minutes

Servings: 2

Ingredients:

- 2 cups cooked chicken, chopped

- 2 medium carrots, chopped

- ½ cup onion, chopped

- ¼ cup lemon juice

- 1 clove garlic, minced

- 1 can cream of chicken soup, fat-free and low sodium

- 2 cans chicken broth, fat-free

- ¼ teaspoon ground black pepper

- 2/3 cup long-grain rice

- 2 tablespoons parsley, snipped

Directions:

1. Add all of the listed ingredients to a pot (except rice and parsley).

2. Season with sunflower seeds and pepper.

3. Bring the mix to a boil over medium-high heat.

4. Stir in rice and set heat to medium.

5. Simmer for 20 minutes until rice is tender.

6. Garnish with parsley and enjoy!

Nutrition:

Calories: 582

Fat: 33g

Carbohydrates: 35g

Protein: 32g

Butternut and Garlic Soup

Preparation Time: 5 minutes

Cooking Time: 35 minutes

Servings: 2

Ingredients:

- 4 cups butternut squash, cubed

- 4 cups vegetable broth, stock

- ½ cup low fat cream

- 2 garlic cloves, chopped

- Pepper to taste

Directions:

1. Add butternut squash, garlic cloves, broth, and pepper in a large pot.

2. Place the pot over medium heat and cover with the lid.

3. Bring to boil and then reduce the temperature.

4. Let it simmer for 30-35 minutes.

5. Blend the soup for 1-2 minutes until you get a smooth mixture.

6. Stir the cream through the soup.

7. Serve and enjoy!

Nutrition:

Calories: 180

Fat: 14g

Carbohydrates: 21g

Protein: 3g

Dinner

Vegetarian Ideas

Cauliflower Steaks with Olive Citrus Sauce

Preparation Time: 15 Minutes

Cooking Time: 30 Minutes

Servings: 2

Ingredients:

- 1 or 2 large heads cauliflower (at least 1 pound, enough for 2 portions)

- ⅓ cup extra-virgin olive oil

- ⅛ teaspoon ground black pepper

- Juice of 1 orange

- Zest of 1 orange

- ¼ cup black olives, pitted and chopped

- 1 tablespoon Dijon or grainy mustard

- 1 tablespoon red wine vinegar

- ½ teaspoon ground coriander

Directions:

1. Preheat the oven to 400°F. Line a baking sheet with parchment paper or foil.

2. Cut off the stem of the cauliflower so it will sit upright. Slice it vertically into four thick slabs. Place the cauliflower on the prepared baking sheet. Drizzle with the olive oil and black pepper. Bake for about 30 minutes, turning over once, until tender and golden brown.

3. In a medium bowl, combine the orange juice, orange zest, olives, mustard, vinegar, and coriander; mix well.

4. Serve the cauliflower warm or at room temperature with the sauce.

Nutrition: Calories: 265; Total fat: 21g; Saturated fat: 3g; Cholesterol: 0mg; Sodium: 310mg; Potassium: 810mg; Total Carbohydrates: 19g; Fiber: 4g; Sugars: 10g; Protein: 5g; Magnesium: 42mg; Calcium: 60mg

Baked Tofu with Sun-Dried Tomatoes and Artichokes

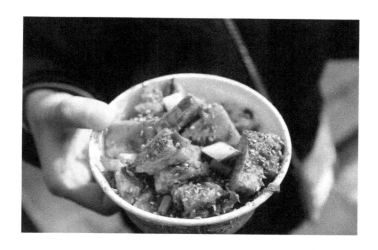

Preparation Time: 15 Minutes, PLUS 15 Minutes TO MARINATE

Cooking Time: 30 Minutes

Servings: 2

Ingredients:

- 1 (16-ounce) package extra-firm tofu, drained and patted dry, cut into 1-inch cubes

- 2 tablespoons extra-virgin olive oil, divided

- 2 tablespoons lemon juice, divided

- 1 tablespoon low-sodium soy sauce or gluten-free tamari

- 1 onion, diced

- 2 garlic cloves, minced

- 1 (14-ounce) can artichoke hearts, drained

- 8 sun-dried tomato halves packed in oil, drained and chopped

- ¼ teaspoon freshly ground black pepper

- 1 tablespoon white wine vinegar

- Zest of 1 lemon

- ¼ cup fresh parsley, chopped

Directions:

1. Preheat the oven to 400°F. Line a baking sheet with foil or parchment paper.

2. In a bowl, combine the tofu, 1 tablespoon of the olive oil, 1 tablespoon of the lemon juice, and the soy sauce. Allow to sit and marinate for 15 to 30 minutes. Arrange the tofu in a

single layer on the prepared baking sheet and bake for 20 minutes, turning once, until light golden brown.

3. Heat the remaining 1 tablespoon olive oil in a large skillet or sauté pan over medium heat.

4. Add the onion and sauté until translucent, 5 to 6 minutes. Add the garlic and sauté for 30 seconds. Add the artichoke hearts, sun-dried tomatoes, and black pepper and sauté for 5 minutes. Add the white wine vinegar and the remaining 1 tablespoon lemon juice and deglaze the pan, scraping up any brown bits. Remove the pan from the heat and stir in the lemon zest and parsley. Gently mix in the baked tofu.

Nutrition: Calories: 230; Total fat: 14g; Saturated fat: 2g; Cholesterol: 0mg; Sodium: 500mg; Potassium: 220mg; Total Carbohydrates: 13g; Fiber: 5g; Sugars: 3g; Protein: 14g; Magnesium: 13mg; Calcium: 110mg

Baked Mediterranean Tempeh with Tomatoes and Garlic

Preparation Time: 25 Minutes, PLUS 4 HOURS TO MARINATE

Cooking Time: 35 Minutes

Servings: 2

Ingredients:

FOR THE TEMPEH

- 12 ounces tempeh

- ¼ cup white wine

- 2 tablespoons extra-virgin olive oil

- 2 tablespoons lemon juice

- Zest of 1 lemon

- ¼ teaspoon freshly ground black pepper

FOR THE TOMATOES AND GARLIC SAUCE

- 1 tablespoon extra-virgin olive oil

- 1 onion, diced

- 3 garlic cloves, minced

- 1 (14.5-ounce) can no-salt-added crushed tomatoes

- 1 beefsteak tomato, diced

- 1 dried bay leaf

- 1 teaspoon white wine vinegar

- 1 teaspoon lemon juice

- 1 teaspoon dried oregano

- 1 teaspoon dried thyme

- ¼ cup basil, cut into ribbons

Directions:

TO MAKE THE TEMPEH

1. Place the tempeh in a medium saucepan. Add enough water to cover it by 1 to 2 inches. Bring to a boil over medium-high heat, cover, and lower heat to a simmer. Cook for 10 to 15 minutes. Remove the tempeh, pat dry, cool, and cut into 1-inch cubes.

2. In a large bowl, combine the white wine, olive oil, lemon juice, lemon zest, and black pepper. Add the tempeh, cover the bowl, and put in the refrigerator for 4 hours, or up to overnight.

3. Preheat the oven to 375°F. Place the marinated tempeh and the marinade in a baking dish and cook for 15 minutes.

TO MAKE THE TOMATOES AND GARLIC SAUCE

4. Heat the olive oil in a large skillet over medium heat. Add the onion and sauté until transparent, 3 to 5 minutes. Add the garlic and sauté for 30 seconds. Add the crushed tomatoes, beefsteak tomato, bay leaf, vinegar, lemon juice, oregano, and thyme. Mix well. Simmer for 15 minutes.

5. Add the baked tempeh to the tomato mixture and gently mix together. Garnish with the basil.

Nutrition: Calories: 330; Total fat: 20g; Saturated fat: 3g; Cholesterol: 0mg; Sodium: 305mg; Potassium: 865mg; Total Carbohydrates: 22g; Fiber: 4g; Sugars: 6g; Protein: 18g; Magnesium: 82mg; Calcium: 125mg

Balsamic Marinated Tofu with Basil and Oregano

Preparation Time: 10 Minutes, PLUS 30 Minutes TO MARINATE

Cooking Time: 30 Minutes

Servings: 2

Ingredients:

- ¼ cup extra-virgin olive oil

- ¼ cup balsamic vinegar

- 2 tablespoons low-sodium soy sauce or gluten-free tamari

- 3 garlic cloves, grated

- 2 teaspoons pure maple syrup

- Zest of 1 lemon

- 1 teaspoon dried basil

- 1 teaspoon dried oregano

- ½ teaspoon dried thyme

- ½ teaspoon dried sage

- ¼ teaspoon freshly ground black pepper

- ¼ teaspoon red pepper flakes (optional)

- 1 (16-ounce) block extra firm tofu, drained and patted dry, cut into ½-inch or 1-inch cubes

Directions:

1. In a bowl or gallon zip-top bag, mix together the olive oil, vinegar, soy sauce, garlic, maple syrup, lemon zest, basil, oregano, thyme, sage, black pepper, and red pepper flakes, if desired. Add the tofu and mix gently. Put in the refrigerator and marinate for 30 minutes, or up to overnight if you desire.

2. Preheat the oven to 425°F. Line a baking sheet with parchment paper or foil. Arrange the marinated tofu in a single layer on the prepared baking sheet. Bake for 20 to 30 minutes, turning over halfway through, until slightly crispy on the outside and tender on the inside.

Nutrition: Calories: 225; Total fat: 16g; Saturated fat: 2g; Cholesterol: 0mg; Sodium: 265mg; Potassium: 65mg; Total Carbohydrates: 9g; Fiber: 2g; Sugars: 5g; Protein: 13g; Magnesium: 6mg; Calcium: 112mg

Poultry Ideas

Creamy Turkey Mix

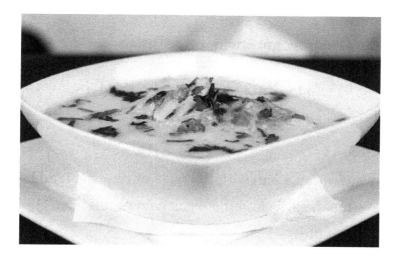

Preparation time: 5 minutes

Cooking time: 25 minutes

Servings: 2

Ingredients:

- 2 tablespoons olive oil

- 1 turkey breast, skinless, boneless and sliced

- A pinch of black pepper

- 1 tablespoon basil, chopped

- 3 garlic cloves, minced

- 14 ounces canned artichokes, no-salt-added, chopped

- 1 cup coconut cream

- ¾ cup low-fat mozzarella, shredded

Directions:

1. Heat up a pan with the oil over high heat, add the meat, garlic and the black pepper, toss and cook for 5 minutes.

2. Add the rest of the ingredients except the cheese, toss and cook over medium heat for 15 minutes.

3. Sprinkle the cheese, cook everything for 5 minutes more, divide between plates and serve.

Nutrition: 268 calories, 8.8g protein, 15g carbohydrates, 21.5g fat, 7.3g fiber, 3mg cholesterol, 225mg sodium, 537mg potassium

Turkey and Onion Mix

Preparation time: 10 minutes

Cooking time: 30 minutes

Servings: 2

Ingredients:

- 2 tablespoons avocado oil

- 1 red onion, chopped

- 2 garlic cloves, minced

- A pinch of black pepper

- 1 tablespoon oregano, chopped

- 1 big turkey breast, skinless, boneless and cubed

- 1 and ½ cups low-sodium beef stock

- 1 tablespoon chives, chopped

Directions:

1. Heat up a pan with the oil over medium heat, and then add the onion, stir and sauté for 3 minutes.

2. Add the garlic and the meat, toss and cook for 3 minutes more.

3. Add the rest of the ingredients, toss, simmer everything over medium heat for 25 minutes, divide between plates and serve.

Nutrition: 32 calories, 1.4g protein, 4.6g carbohydrates, 1.1g fat, 1.4g fiber, 0mg cholesterol, 154mg sodium, 90mg potassium

Balsamic Chicken

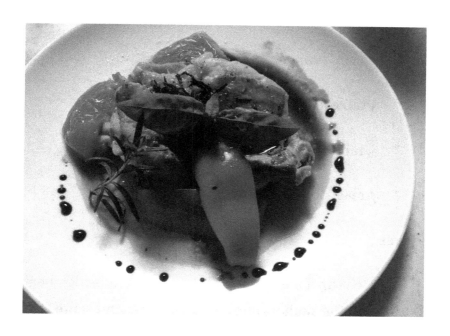

Preparation time: 10 minutes

Cooking time: 35 minutes

Servings: 2

Ingredients:

- 1 tablespoon avocado oil

- 1 pound chicken breast, skinless, boneless and halved

- 2 garlic cloves, minced

- 2 shallots, chopped

- ½ cup orange juice

- 1 tablespoon orange zest, grated

- 3 tablespoons balsamic vinegar

- 1 teaspoon rosemary, chopped

Directions:

1. Heat up a pan with the oil over medium-high heat; add the shallots and the garlic, toss and sauté for 2 minutes.

2. Add the meat, toss gently and cook for 3 minutes more.

3. Add the rest of the ingredients, toss, introduce the pan in the oven and bake at 340 degrees F for 30 minutes.

4. Divide between plates and serve.

Nutrition: 159 calories, 24.6g protein, 5.4g carbohydrates, 3.4g fat, 0.5g fiber, 73mg cholesterol, 60mg sodium, 530mg potassium

Turkey and Garlic Sauce

Preparation time: 10 minutes

Cooking time: 40 minutes

Servings: 2

Ingredients:

- 1 turkey breast, boneless, skinless and cubed

- ½ pound white mushrooms, halved

- 1/3 cup coconut aminos

- 2 garlic cloves, minced

- 2 tablespoons olive oil

- A pinch of black pepper

- 2 green onion, chopped

- 3 tablespoons garlic sauce

- 1 tablespoon rosemary, chopped

Directions:

1. Heat up a pan with the oil over medium heat; add the green onions, garlic sauce and the garlic and sauté for 5 minutes.

2. Add the meat and brown it for 5 minutes more.

3. Add the rest of the ingredients, introduce in the oven and bake at 390 degrees F for 30 minutes.

4. Divide the mix between plates and serve.

Nutrition: 100 calories, 2.1g protein, 7.5g carbohydrates, 7.3g fat, 1.2g fiber, 0mg cholesterol, 30mg sodium, 216mg potassium

Basil Turkey and Broccoli

Preparation time: 10 minutes

Cooking time: 25 minutes

Servings: 2

Ingredients:

- 1 tablespoon olive oil

- 1 big turkey breast, skinless, boneless and cubed

- 2 cups broccoli florets

- 2 shallots, chopped

- 2 garlic cloves, minced

- 1 tablespoon basil, chopped

- 1 tablespoon cilantro, chopped

- ½ cup coconut cream

Directions:

1. Heat up a pan with the oil over medium-high heat, after that, add the meat, shallots and the garlic, toss and brown for 5 minutes.

2. Add the broccoli and the other ingredients, toss everything, cook for 20 minutes over medium heat, divide between plates and serve.

Nutrition: 121 calories, 2.3g protein, 6.1g carbohydrates, 10.8g fat, 1.9g fiber, 0mg cholesterol, 23mg sodium, 250mg potassium

Chicken with Zucchini

Preparation time: 5 minutes

Cooking time: 25 minutes

Servings: 2

Ingredients:

- 1 pound chicken breasts, skinless, boneless and cubed

- 1 cup low-sodium chicken stock

- 2 zucchinis, roughly cubed

- 1 tablespoon olive oil

- 1 cup canned tomatoes, no-salt-added, chopped

- 1 yellow onion, chopped

- 1 teaspoon chili powder

- 1 tablespoon cilantro, chopped

Directions:

1. Heat up a pan with the oil over medium heat, add the meat and the onion, toss and brown it for about 5 minutes.

2. Add the zucchinis and the rest of the ingredients toss gently, reduce the heat to medium and cook for 20 minutes.

3. Divide everything between plates and serve.

Nutrition: 284 calories, 35g protein, 14.8g carbohydrates, 8g fat, 12.3g fiber, 2.4mg cholesterol, 151mg sodium, 693mg potassium

Ginger Turkey Mix

Preparation time: 10 minutes

Cooking time: 20 minutes

Servings: 2

Ingredients:

- 1 turkey breast, boneless, skinless and roughly cubed

- 2 scallions, chopped

- 1 pound bok choy, torn

- 2 tablespoons olive oil

- ½ teaspoon ginger, grated

- A pinch of black pepper

- ½ cup low-sodium vegetable stock

Directions:

1. Heat up a pot with the oil over medium-high heat; add the scallions and the ginger and sauté for 2 minutes.

2. Add the meat and brown for 5 minutes more.

3. Add the rest of the ingredients, toss, simmer for 13 minutes more, divide between plates and serve.

Nutrition: 81 calories, 2g protein, 3.7g carbohydrates, 7.3g fat, 1.5g fiber, 0mg cholesterol, 95mg sodium, 327mg potassium

Chives Chicken

Preparation time: 10 minutes

Cooking time: 25 minutes

Servings: 2

Ingredients:

- 2 chicken breasts, skinless, boneless and roughly cubed

- 3 red onions, sliced

- 2 tablespoons olive oil

- 1 cup low-sodium vegetable stock

- A pinch of black pepper

- 1 tablespoon cilantro, chopped

- 1 tablespoon chives, chopped

Directions:

1. Heat up a pan with the oil over medium heat; add the onions and a pinch of black pepper, and sauté for 10 minutes stirring often.

2. Add the chicken and cook for 3 minutes more.

3. Add the rest of the ingredients, bring it to a simmer and cook over medium heat for 12 minutes more.

4. Divide the chicken and onions mix between plates and serve.

Nutrition: 99 calories, 1.3g protein, 8.8g carbohydrates, 7.1g fat, 2.1g fiber, 0mg cholesterol, 39mg sodium, 158mg potassium

Turkey with Pepper and Rice

Preparation time: 10 minutes

Cooking time: 42 minutes

Servings: 2

Ingredients:

- 1 turkey breast, skinless, boneless and cubed

- 1 cup white rice

- 2 cups low-sodium vegetable stock

- 1 teaspoon hot paprika

- 2 small Serrano peppers, chopped

- 2 garlic cloves, minced

- 2 tablespoons olive oil

- ½ red bell pepper chopped

- A pinch of black pepper

Directions:

1. Heat up a pan with the oil over medium heat; add the Serrano peppers and garlic and sauté for 2 minutes.

2. Add the meat and brown it for 5 minutes.

3. Add the rice and the other ingredients bring to a simmer and cook over medium heat for 35 minutes.

4. Stir, divide between plates and serve.

Nutrition: 245 calories, 4g protein, 40.2g carbohydrates, 7.3g fat, 1.3g fiber, 0mg cholesterol, 76mg sodium, 134mg potassium

Meat Ideas

Cilantro Pork

Preparation time: 10 minutes

Cooking time: 35 minutes

Servings: 2

Ingredients:

- 2 red onions, sliced

- 2 green onions, chopped

- 1 tablespoon olive oil

- 2 teaspoons ginger, grated

- 4 pork chops

- 3 garlic cloves, chopped

- Black pepper to the taste

- 1 carrot, chopped

- 1 cup low sodium beef stock

- 2 tablespoons tomato paste

- 1 tablespoon cilantro, chopped

Directions:

1. Heat up a pan with the oil over medium heat, add the green and red onions, toss and sauté them for 3 minutes.

2. Add the garlic and the ginger, toss and cook for 2 minutes more.

3. Add the pork chops and cook them for 2 minutes on each side.

4. Add the rest of the ingredients and bring to a simmer and cook over medium heat for 25 minutes more.

5. Divide the mix between plates and serve.

Nutrition: 332 calories, 19.9g protein, 10.1g carbohydrates, 23.6g fat, 2.3g fiber, 69mg cholesterol, 11mg sodium, 528mg potassium

Coriander Pork

Preparation time: 10 minutes

Cooking time: 45 minutes

Servings: 2

Ingredients:

- ½ cup low-sodium beef stock

- 2 tablespoons olive oil

- 2 pounds pork stew meat, cubed

- 1 teaspoon coriander, ground

- 2 teaspoons cumin, ground

- Black pepper to the taste

- 1 cup cherry tomatoes, halved

- 4 garlic cloves, minced

- 1 tablespoon cilantro, chopped

Directions:

1. Heat up a pan with the oil over medium heat, add the garlic and the meat, toss and brown for 5 minutes.

2. Add the stock and the other ingredients bring to a simmer and cook over medium heat for 40 minutes.

3. Divide everything between plates and serve.

Nutrition: 559 calories, 67.4g protein, 10.1g carbohydrates, 3.2g fat, 29.3g fiber, 195mg cholesterol, 156mg sodium, 988mg potassium

Lamb and Cherry Tomatoes Mix

Preparation time: 10 minutes

Cooking time: 25 minutes

Servings: 2

Ingredients:

- 1 tablespoon olive oil

- 1 red onion, chopped

- 1 cup cherry tomatoes, halved

- 1 pound lamb stew meat, ground

- 1 tablespoon chili powder

- Black pepper to the taste

- 2 teaspoons cumin, ground

- 1 cup low-sodium vegetable stock

- 2 tablespoons cilantro, chopped

Directions:

1. Heat up the a pan with the oil over medium-high heat, add the onion, lamb and chili powder, toss and cook for 10 minutes.

2. Add the rest of the ingredients, toss, and cook over medium heat for 15 minutes more.

3. Divide into bowls and serve.

Nutrition: 275 calories, 33.2g protein, 6.8g carbohydrates, 12.5g fat, 2.1g fiber, 102mg cholesterol, 145mg sodium, 617mg potassium

Balsamic Pork

Preparation time: 10 minutes

Cooking time: 20 minutes

Servings: 2

Ingredients:

- 2 tablespoons balsamic vinegar

- 1/3 cup coconut aminos

- 1 tablespoon olive oil

- 4 ounces mixed salad greens

- 1 cup cherry tomatoes, halved

- 4 ounces pork stew meat, cut into strips

- 1 tablespoon chives, chopped

Directions:

1. Heat up a pan with the oil over medium heat, add the pork, coconut aminos and the vinegar, toss and cook for 15 minutes.

2. Add the salad greens and the other ingredients, toss, cook for 5 minutes more, divide between plates and serve.

Nutrition: 125 calories, 9.1g protein, 6.8g carbohydrates, 6.4g fat, 0.6g fiber, 24mg cholesterol, 49mg sodium, 269mg potassium

Cilantro Pork Skillet

Preparation time: 10 minutes

Cooking time: 25 minutes

Servings: 2

Ingredients:

- 1 pound pork butt, trimmed and cubed

- 1 tablespoon olive oil

- 1 yellow onion, chopped

- 3 garlic cloves, minced

- 1 tablespoon thyme, dried

- 1 cup low-sodium chicken stock

- 2 tablespoons low-sodium tomato paste

- 1 tablespoon cilantro, chopped

Directions:

1. Heat up a pan with the oil over medium-high heat, add the onion and the garlic, toss and cook for 5 minutes.

2. Add the meat, toss and cook for 5 more minutes.

3. Add the rest of the ingredients, toss, bring to a simmer, reduce heat to medium and cook the mix for 15 minutes more.

4. Divide the mix between plates and serve right away.

Nutrition: 274 calories, 36.6g protein, 5.3g carbohydrates, 11.2g fat, 1.2g fiber, 104mg cholesterol, 104mg sodium, 484mg potassium

Pork and Zucchinis

Preparation time: 10 minutes

Cooking time: 30 minutes

Servings: 2

Ingredients:

- 2 pounds pork loin boneless, trimmed and cubed

- 2 tablespoons avocado oil

- ¾ cup low-sodium vegetable stock

- ½ tablespoon garlic powder

- 1 tablespoon marjoram, chopped

- 2 zucchinis, roughly cubed

- 1 teaspoon sweet paprika

- Black pepper to the taste

Directions:

1. Heat up a pan with the oil over medium-high heat

2. Add the meat, garlic powder and the marjoram, toss and cook for 10 minutes.

3. Add the zucchinis and the other ingredients toss, bring it to a simmer, reduce heat to medium and cook the mix for 20 minutes more.

4. Divide everything between plates and serve.

Nutrition: 359 calories, 61.1g protein, 5.7g carbohydrates, 9.1g fat, 2.1g fiber, 166mg cholesterol, 166mg sodium, 1289mg potassium

Peppercorn Pork

Preparation time: 10 minutes

Cooking time: 35 minutes

Servings: 2

Ingredients:

- 2 pounds pork stew meat, cubed

- 2 tablespoons olive oil

- 1 cup low-sodium vegetable stock

- 1 celery stalk, chopped

- 1 teaspoon black peppercorns

- 2 shallots, chopped

- 1 tablespoon chives, chopped

- 1 cup coconut cream

Directions:

1. Heat up a pan with the oil over medium heat, add the shallots and the meat, toss and brown for 5 minutes.

2. Add the celery and the other ingredients toss bring to a simmer and cook over medium heat for 30 minutes more.

3. Divide everything between plates and serve right away.

Nutrition: 690 calories, 68.2g protein, 5.7g carbohydrates, 43.3g fat, 1.8g fiber, 195mg cholesterol, 182mg sodium, 1077mg potassium

Parsley Pork and Tomatoes

Preparation time: 10 minutes

Cooking time: 30 minutes

Servings: 2

Ingredients:

- 2 garlic cloves, minced

- 2 pounds pork stew meat, ground

- 2 cups cherry tomatoes, halved

- 1 tablespoon olive oil

- Black pepper to the taste

- 1 red onion, chopped

- ½ cup low-sodium vegetable stock

- 2 tablespoons low-sodium tomato paste

- 1 tablespoon parsley, chopped

Directions:

1. Heat up a pan with the oil over medium heat; add the onion and the garlic, toss and sauté for 5 minutes.

2. Add the meat and brown it for 5 minutes more.

3. Add the rest of the ingredients, toss, bring to a simmer, cook over medium heat for 20 minutes more, divide into bowls and serve.

Nutrition: 551 calories, 68.2g protein, 8.6g carbohydrates, 25.6g fat, 2.1g fiber, 195mg cholesterol, 163mg sodium, 1131mg potassium

Lemon Pork Chops

Preparation time: 10 minutes

Cooking time: 35 minutes

Servings: 2

Ingredients:

- 4 pork chops

- 2 tablespoons olive oil

- 1 teaspoon smoked paprika

- 1 tablespoon sage, chopped

- 2 garlic cloves, minced

- 1 tablespoon lemon juice

- Black pepper to the taste

Directions:

1. In a baking dish, combine the pork chops with the oil and the other ingredients, toss, introduce in the oven and bake at 400 degrees F for 35 minutes.

2. Divide the pork chops between plates and serve with a side salad.

Nutrition: 322 calories, 18.2g protein, 1.2g carbohydrates, 27.1g fat, 0.5g fiber, 69mg cholesterol, 57mg sodium, 304mg potassium

Lamb Chops and Greens

Preparation time: 10 minutes

Cooking time: 35 minutes

Servings: 2

Ingredients:

- 1 cup kale, torn

- 1 pound lamb chops

- ½ cup low-sodium vegetable stock

- 2 tablespoons low-sodium tomato paste

- 1 yellow onion, sliced

- 1 tablespoon olive oil

- A pinch of black pepper

Directions:

1. Grease a roasting pan with the oil, arrange the lamb chops inside, also add the kale and the other ingredients and toss gently.

2. Bake everything at 390 degrees F for 35 minutes, divide between plates and serve.

Nutrition: 270calories, 33.3g protein, 6.3g carbohydrates, 11.8g fat, 1.2g fiber, 102mg cholesterol, 117mg sodium, 519mg potassium

Fish And Seafood Ideas

Tex-Mex Cod with Roasted Peppers & Corn

Preparation Time: 10 Minutes

Cooking Time: 30 Minutes

Servings: 2

Ingredients:

- 6 mini bell peppers, assorted colors, quartered

- 1 cup frozen corn

- 2 teaspoons olive oil, divided

- 1 tablespoon salt-free Tex-Mex or mesquite seasoning, divided

- Nonstick cooking spray

- 2 (6- to 8-ounce) haddock fillets

- 1 lime, quartered

- ¼ cup plain Greek yogurt, seasoned with ¼ teaspoon salt-free Tex-Mex seasoning (optional)

Directions:

1. Preheat the oven to 425°F. Line a baking sheet with parchment paper or a silicone mat.

2. Spread the peppers and corn evenly over two-thirds of the baking sheet. Drizzle 1 teaspoon of oil over the vegetables, and then sprinkle them with 2 teaspoons of the seasoning. Put the vegetables in the oven for 10 minutes to begin roasting. Remove baking sheet from the oven.

3. While the vegetables roast, spray a sheet of aluminum foil with cooking spray and place the fish on it. Drizzle the fish with the remaining oil and season it with the remaining 1 teaspoon of seasoning. Squeeze one lime wedge onto each fillet. Fold up the edges of the foil so the juices don't escape and transfer the fish to the baking sheet with the vegetables.

4. Return the baking sheet to the oven and bake for an additional 15 to 20 minutes until the fish is opaque white and flaky and the vegetables are tender and lightly charred.

5. Place a fish fillet on each plate, and top each with half of the roasted vegetables. Serve with a dollop of seasoned yogurt (if using).

Nutrition: Calories: 340; Total fat: 7g; Carbohydrates: 38g; Fiber: 5g; Protein: 36g; Calcium: 84mg; Sodium: 382mg; Potassium: 1316mg; Vitamin D: 1mcg; Iron: 2mg; Zinc: 2mg

Marinated Lime Grilled Shrimp

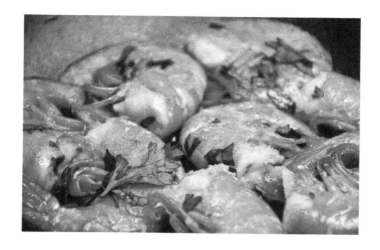

Preparation Time: 10 Minutes, PLUS AT LEAST 30 Minutes TO MARINATE

Cooking Time: 10 Minutes

Servings: 2

Ingredients:

- 1 lime, quartered, divided

- ¼ cup chopped fresh cilantro, divided

- 1 tablespoon rice wine vinegar

- 1 teaspoon avocado oil

- ¼ teaspoon chili powder

- ¼ teaspoon garlic powder

- 6 large shrimp, peeled and deveined

Directions:

1. In a small bowl, mix together the juice from three lime quarters, 3 tablespoons cilantro, and the vinegar, oil, chili powder, and garlic powder.

2. Place the shrimp in the bowl with the marinade, toss to coat, and refrigerate it for 30 minutes or up to 4 hours.

3. Preheat a grill to medium-high. Place the shrimp on a grill pan and cook for 3 to 5 minutes, until white, turning once. Discard the marinade.

4. If you do not have a grill, pan-sear the shrimp in a nonstick skillet for 3 to 4 minutes, turning once.

5. Serve the shrimp with a squeeze of juice from the last lime quarter and the remaining cilantro.

Nutrition: Calories: 44; Total fat: 2g; Carbohydrates: 3g; Fiber: 0g; Protein: 3g; Calcium: 18mg; Sodium: 131mg; Potassium: 74mg; Vitamin D: 0mcg; Iron: 0 mg; Zinc: 0mg

Bass with Citrus Butter

Preparation Time: 15 Minutes

Cooking Time: 15 Minutes

Servings: 2

Ingredients:

- 2 (5- to 7-ounce) bass fillets, skin-on

- 1 teaspoon salt-free seafood seasoning

- 1 lime, halved

- 1 tablespoon avocado oil, divided

- 1 teaspoon butter

- ¼ teaspoon cumin

- ¼ cup slivered, blanched almonds

Directions:

1. Season the fish with the seasoning blend.

2. In a microwave-safe glass measuring cup, stir together the juice of half a lime, 2 teaspoons oil, butter, and cumin until blended. Set aside.

3. Heat a large nonstick skillet over medium heat. Add the almonds and toast for 2 to 3 minutes, being careful they don't over-brown. Transfer the almonds to a small bowl and set aside.

4. Heat the remaining oil in the skillet over medium-high heat. Add the bass fillets, skin side up. Sear for 3 minutes without disturbing the fillets, then turn them and finish cooking for another 3 to 4 minutes.

5. While the fish is searing, heat the citrus butter sauce for 20 seconds in the microwave.

6. Transfer the fish to a serving dish, pour the citrus butter over it, and top it with the toasted almonds. Garnish with the remaining lime half cut into wedges and serve.

Nutrition: Calories: 325; Total fat: 21g; Carbohydrates: 5g; Fiber: 2g; Protein: 30g; Calcium: 156mg; Sodium: 270mg; Potassium: 634mg; Vitamin D: 13mcg; Iron: 3mg; Zinc: 1mg

Seared Mahi-Mahi with Lemon & Parsley

Preparation Time: 20 Minutes, PLUS AT LEAST 15 Minutes TO MARINATE

Cooking Time: 15 Minutes

Servings: 2

Ingredients:

- 2 teaspoons avocado oil

- Juice of ½ lemon

- ½ teaspoon oregano

- ½ teaspoon garlic powder

- ¼ teaspoon Worcestershire sauce

- 2 (5- to 7-ounce) mahi-mahi steaks

- 1 tablespoon chopped parsley

- ½ lemon, cut into two wedges

Directions:

1. Preheat the oven to 400°F. (If you'll be marinating the fish for longer than 15 minutes, preheat the oven just before baking.) Line a baking sheet with parchment paper or a silicone mat.

2. In a medium bowl, stir together the oil, lemon juice, oregano, garlic powder, and Worcestershire sauce. Put the fish in a medium zip-top plastic bag and add the marinade. Press out any excess air, seal the bag, and marinate the fish in the refrigerator for 15 minutes or up to 2 hours.

3. Remove the fish from the marinade, place it on the prepared baking sheet, and roast it for 15 minutes (discard the marinade).

4. To serve, garnish each mahi-mahi steak with parsley and a lemon wedge.

Nutrition: Calories: 282; Total fat: 18g; Carbohydrates: 3g; Fiber: g; Protein: 26g; Calcium: 41mg; Sodium: 101mg; Potassium: 594mg; Vitamin D: 16mcg; Iron: 1mg; Zinc: 1mg

Pan-Fried Crusted Salmon with Mustard Panko

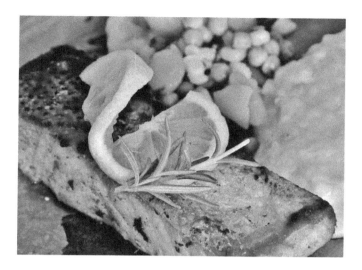

Preparation Time: 5 Minutes

Cooking Time: 10 Minutes

Servings: 2

Ingredients:

- 1 tablespoon Dijon mustard

- 1 tablespoon light sour cream

- 2 skinless salmon fillets (5 to 6 ounces each)

- ¼ cup panko bread crumbs

- ½ teaspoon salt-free mesquite seasoning

- 1 teaspoon olive oil

- 1 teaspoon unsalted butter

Directions:

1. In a small bowl, combine the mustard and sour cream. Spread the mustard mixture onto both sides of each salmon fillet, dividing evenly between the two.

2. Mix the panko bread crumbs and seasoning together in a small bowl. Press each fillet into the seasoned crumbs, lightly coating both sides.

3. Heat the oil and butter in a large nonstick skillet over medium-high heat. Place the fish into the hot fat to fry. Gently turn each fillet after 4 to 5 minutes, and pan-fry the other side for another 5 to 6 minutes until lightly browned. The salmon should change to a lighter color but not be opaque. Serve hot.

Nutrition: Calories: 307; Total fat: 15g; Carbohydrates: 11g; Fiber: 1g; Protein: 31g; Calcium: 56mg; Sodium: 689mg; Potassium: 746mg; Vitamin D: 9mcg; Iron: 2mg; Zinc: 1mg

Seared Ginger–Soy Ahi Tuna

Preparation Time: 10 Minutes

Cooking Time: 2 Minutes

Servings: 2

Ingredients:

- 2 tablespoons reduced-sodium soy sauce, divided

- Juice of 1 lime

- 2 teaspoons Dijon mustard

- ¼ teaspoon ground ginger

- 10 ounces sushi-grade tuna

- 1 teaspoon olive oil

- 4 scallions, both white and green parts, thinly sliced

Directions:

1. In a small bowl, mix together 1 tablespoon of the soy sauce with the lime juice, mustard, and ginger until blended. Using a basting brush, brush the mixture onto each side of the tuna.

2. Heat the oil in a large nonstick skillet over high heat. Add the tuna, searing one side for 1 minute. Flip the fish over and sear the other side for 1 minute. The fish should still be pink in the middle.

3. Remove the tuna from the skillet, transfer it to a small serving platter, and cut it on the diagonal into ¼-inch slices. Top with the scallions and serve with the remaining soy sauce.

Nutrition: Calories: 126; Total fat: 5g; Carbohydrates: 3g; Fiber: 1g; Protein: 18g; Calcium: 22mg; Sodium: 313mg; Potassium: 263mg; Vitamin D: 4mcg; Iron: 1mg; Zinc: 1mg

Greek-Style Cod with Olives & Tomatoes

Preparation Time: 15 Minutes

Cooking Time: 35 Minutes

Servings: 2

Ingredients:

- 1 pint grape or cherry tomatoes, halved

- ⅓ cup mixed olives, pitted, roughly chopped

- 1 teaspoon olive oil

- 2 cod fillets (5 to 8 ounces each)

- 1 teaspoon Herbs de Provence

- 2 lemon wedges, for garnish

Directions:

1. Preheat the oven to 375°F. Line a baking sheet with parchment paper or a silicone mat.

2. Place the tomatoes and olives on one half of the baking sheet and drizzle them with olive oil. Roast in the oven for 15 minutes.

3. Remove the baking sheet from the oven, place the cod fillets on the empty side, and season both the tomato mixture and the fish with Herbs de Provence. Bake for 15 to 20 minutes until the fish is opaque.

4. Serve the fish topped with the olive-tomato mixture and garnished with a squeeze of lemon.

Nutrition: Calories: 186; Total fat: 6g; Carbohydrates: 8g; Fiber: 2g; Protein: 26g; Calcium: 53mg; Sodium: 244mg; Potassium: 813mg; Vitamin D: 1mcg; Iron: 2mg; Zinc: 1mg

Pesto Tilapia

Preparation Time: 5 Minutes

Cooking Time: 20 Minutes

Servings: 2

Ingredients:

- ¼ cup dry white wine

- 1 teaspoon avocado oil

- 1 lemon, halved

- 2 tilapia fillets (5 to 7 ounces each)

- Freshly ground black pepper

- 2 tablespoons store-bought low-sodium pesto

Directions:

1. Preheat the oven to 350°F.

2. In a 9-by-11-inch baking dish, whisk the wine, oil, and juice of half a lemon. Add the fish fillets and season lightly with pepper.

3. Cover the baking dish with foil and bake for 15 minutes. Uncover the dish, top each fillet with 1 tablespoon pesto, and cook for 5 more minutes.

4. Cut the remaining ½ lemon into wedges and serve each fillet with a lemon wedge.

Nutrition: Calories: 272; Total fat: 13g; Carbohydrates: 3g; Fiber: 0g; Protein: 30g; Calcium: 56mg; Sodium: 220mg; Potassium: 502mg; Vitamin D: 4mcg; Iron: 1mg; Zinc: 1mg

Desserts

Light Choco Pudding

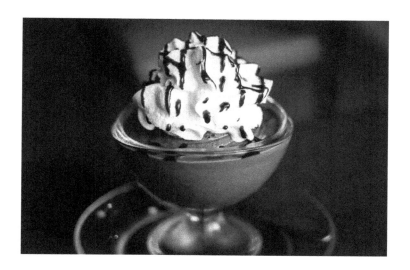

Preparation time: 32 minutes

Cooking time: 12 minutes

Servings: 2

Ingredients:

- 1 teaspoon vanilla extract

- 2 cups chocolate soy milk

- 2 tablespoons baking cocoa

- 2 tablespoons sugar

- 3 tablespoons cornstarch

Directions:

1. Put milk in a pan over medium flame. Add cocoa, sugar, and cornstarch. Mix until thick and bubbly. Turn heat to low and continue cooking for 2 minutes.

2. Turn off the heat, add vanilla and allow to cool while stirring every now and then. Transfer to a bowl, cover and refrigerate for 30 minutes before serving.

Nutrition:

Calories: 127

Protein: 4.38 g

Fat: 1.49 g

Carbohydrates: 27.14 g

Sodium: 112 mg

Peach Tart

Preparation time: 20 minutes

Cooking time: 52 minutes

Servings: 2

Ingredients:

- 1 cup all-purpose flour

- 1/4 teaspoon ground nutmeg

- 3 tablespoons sugar

- 1/4 cup butter (softened)

For the filling:

- 1/4 cup sliced almonds

- 1/8 teaspoon almond extract

- 1/4 teaspoon ground cinnamon

- Whipped cream (optional)

- 2 tablespoons all-purpose flour

- 1/3 cup sugar

- 2 pounds peaches (peeled and sliced)

Directions:

1. Put butter, sugar, and butter in a bowl. Mix until fluffy. Add flour and beat until combined. Transfer to a tart pan and firmly spread and press to the bottom. Put on a baking sheet in the oven's middle rack. Bake in a preheated oven at 375 degrees F for 12 minutes. Leave to cool.

2. Put peaches in a bowl. Add almond extract, cinnamon, flour, and sugar. Toss to coat. Scoop on top of the crust. Add chopped almonds on top. Put on the lower rack of the oven and bake for 40 minutes. Allow to cool.

3. Serve as is or you can also opt to top it with whipped cream.

Nutrition:

Calories: 222

Protein: 2.61 g , Fat: 6.14 g

Carbohydrates: 47.84 g

Sodium: 46 mg

Fruit and Nut Bites

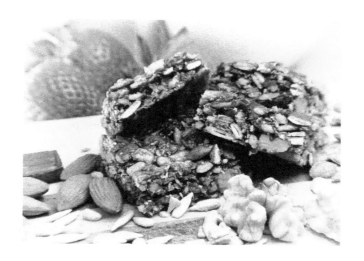

Preparation time: 1 hour

Cooking time: 0 minute

Servings: 2

Ingredients:

- 1 cup pistachios (toasted and finely chopped)

- 1 cup dried cherries (finely chopped)

- 2 cups dried apricots (finely chopped)

- 1/4 cup honey

- 1/4 teaspoon almond extract

- 3 3/4 cups sliced almonds (divided)

Directions:

1. Put 1 1/4 cups of almonds in a food processor. Pulse until chopped. Transfer to a bowl and set aside.

2. Process 2 1/2 cups almonds in a food processor until chopped. Gradually add extract and honey as you process. Transfer to a bowl. Add cherries and apricots. Divide into 6 and shape them into thick rolls. Wrap in plastic and leave in the fridge for an hour.

3. Remove plastic and cut each roll to 1 1/2 inch piece. Roll half of them in pistachios. Roll the other half in almonds. Wrap each piece in waxed paper and store in an airtight container.

Nutrition:

Calories: 86

Protein: 9.22 g , Fat: 14.95 g

Carbohydrates: 72.36 g

Sodium: 15 mg

Tropical Fruit Napoleon

Preparation Time: 20 minutes

Cooking Time: 0 minutes

Servings: 2

Ingredients:

- 1 tbsp. finely chopped fresh lemongrass

- 1 c. cubed mango

- 1 tsp. vanilla extract

- 1 peeled and cored whole pineapple

- 1 c. shredded unsweetened coconut

- 2 c. cubed papaya

- 2 c. light whipping cream

Directions:

1. Add the vanilla extract to the whipping cream and beat until thick and creamy. Fold in the coconut and lemongrass. Place in the refrigerator to chill for at least 30 minutes.

2. Cut the pineapple in thin, lengthwise pieces, creating "sheets" of pineapple.

3. Mix the mango and papaya together in a bowl.

4. Lay one-third of the pineapple sheets on your cake dish.

5. Spread a third of the whipping cream onto the pineapple.

6. Top with some mango and papaya. Follow this with another layer of pineapple, cream, and fruit.

7. Top with a final layer of pineapple, cream, and fruit.

8. Serve chilled and garnish with additional lemongrass, if desired.

Nutrition:

Calories: 128.5

Fat: 6.9 g

Carbs: 17.7 g , Protein: 1.0 g

Sugars: 6 g

Sodium: 80 mg

Ginger Peach Pie

Preparation Time: 10 minutes

Cooking Time: 45 minutes

Servings: 2

Ingredients:

- 5 c. diced peaches

- ½ c. sugar

- 2 refrigerated whole wheat pie crust dough

- 1 tsp. cinnamon

- ½ c. orange juice

- ¼ c. chopped candied ginger

- ½ c. cornstarch

Directions:

1. Preheat the oven to 425°F.

2. Place one of the pie crusts in a standard size pie dish. Spread some coffee beans or dried beans in the bottom of

the pie crust to use as a weight. Place the dish in the oven and bake for 10-15 minutes, or until lightly golden. Remove from the oven and let cool.

3. Combine the peaches, candied ginger, and cinnamon in a bowl. Toss to mix.

4. Combine the sugar, cornstarch, and orange juice in a saucepan and heat over medium until syrup begins to thicken.

5. Pour the syrup over the peaches and toss to coat.

6. Spread the peaches in the pie crust and top with the remaining crust. Crimp along the edges and cut several small slits in the top.

7. Place in the oven and bake for 25-30 minutes, or until golden brown.

8. Let set before slicing.

Nutrition:

Calories: 289.0 , Fat: 13.1 g

Carbs: 41.6 g , Protein: 3.9 g

Sugars: 22 g , Sodium: 154 mg

Apples and Cream Shake

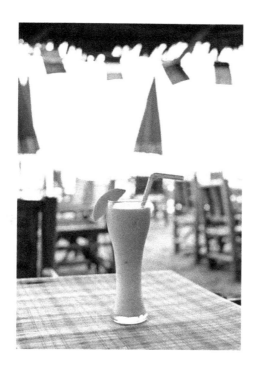

Preparation time: 10 minutes

Cooking time: 0 minutes

Servings: 2

Ingredients:

- 2 cups vanilla low fat ice cream

- 1 cup apple sauce

- 1/4 teaspoon ground cinnamon

- 1 cup fat free skim milk

Directions:

1. In a blender container combine the low fat ice cream, applesauce and cinnamon. Cover and blend until smooth.

2. Add fat free skim milk. Cover and blend until mixed.

3. Pour into glasses.

4. Serve immediately.

5. Nutrition:

Calories 160

Total fat 3 g

Saturated fat 2 g

Carbohydrates 27 g

Protein 6 g

Fiber 1 g

Sodium 80 mg

Potassium 46 mg

Magnesium 2 mg

Calcium 181 mg

Conclusion

Thank you for making it to the end of this cookbook!

I hope that I was able to convey to you how important is in our lives a healthy food regime and how the DASH diet can help you.

The DASH diet is not a typical diet that briefly changes your food habits to achieve a specific goal, such as "losing x pounds". The DASH diet is not just about restricting yourself for a few days or weeks, but rather a long-term change in the way you eat and in the quality of food you choose.

DASH diet inevitably leads to weight loss solely through the conscious consumption of calories, a lower assumption of sodium and a diet with healthy foods.

The diet can be implemented in a few days and the ingredients in the menu plan are simple and common.

I sincerely hope you will be able to implement this diet into your life, quickly and easily, to start enjoying very soon the great improvements the DASH can deliver to you.

I wish you good luck, happiness and health on your path in life!

Photo credits: Thanks to Pixabay

CPSIA information can be obtained
at www.ICGtesting.com
Printed in the USA
BVHW091013280521
608375BV00009B/1247